C000142710

EASY STROKE REHABILITATION EXERCISES FOR THE ENTIRE BODY

AT HOME EXERCISES FOR STROKE SURVIVORS

Dr.Denney Erin

Cover design by VAX Graphix

ISBN: 9798653671883

Published by VAX Books

VaxbookZ.com

TABLE OF CONTENTS

STROKE REHABILITATION EXERCISES FOR YOUR BODY

Stroke survival rates have improved a lot over the last few years. Stroke was once the third leading cause of death in the United States, but it fell to fourth place in 2008 and fifth place in 2013. Today, strokes claim an average of 129,000 American lives every year. Reducing stroke deaths in America is a great improvement, but we still have a long way to go in improving the lives of stroke survivors.

Stagnant recovery rates and low quality of life for stroke survivors are unfortunately very common. Just 10% of stroke survivors make a full recovery. Only 25% of all survivors recover with minor impairments. Nearly half of all stroke survivors continue to live with serious impairments requiring special care, and 10% of survivors live in nursing homes, skilled nursing facilities, and other long-term healthcare facilities. It's easy to see why stroke is the leading cause of long-term disability in the United States. By 2030, it's estimated that there could be up to 11 million stroke survivors in the country.

Traditionally, stroke rehabilitation in America leaves much to be desired in terms of recovery and quality of life. There is a serious gap between stroke patients being discharged and transitioning to physical recovery programs. In an effort to improve recovery and quality of life, the American Heart Association has urged the healthcare community to prioritize exercise as an essential part of post-stroke care.

"There is strong evidence that physical activity and exercise after stroke can improve cardiovascular fitness, walking ability, and upper arm strength. In addition, emerging research suggests exercise may improve depressive symptoms, cognitive function, memory, and quality of life after stroke."

- Sandra Billinger, Physical Therapist at the University of Kansas Medical Center

Unfortunately, too few healthcare professionals prescribe exercise as a form of therapy for stroke, despite its many benefits for patients. Many stroke survivors are not given the skills, confidence, knowledge, or tools necessary to follow an exercise program. However, that can change.

With the right recovery programs that prioritize exercise for rehabilitation, stroke survivors can "relearn" crucial motors skills to regain a high quality of life. Thanks to a phenomenon known as neuroplasticity, even permanent brain damage doesn't make disability inevitable.

HOW YOUR BRAIN RECOVERS FROM A STROKE

A stroke causes loss of physical function because it temporarily or permanently damages the parts of the brain responsible for those functions. The same damage is also responsible for behavioral and cognitive changes, which range from memory and vision problems to severe depression and anger. Each of these changes correspond to a specific region of the brain that was damaged due to stroke.

For example, damage in the left hemisphere of your brain will cause weakness and paralysis on the right side of your body. If a stroke damages or kills brain cells in the right hemisphere, you may struggle to understand facial cues or control your behavior. However, brain damage due to stroke is not necessarily permanent.

Even when brain cells are destroyed completely, recovery is still possible because the human brain is capable of reorganizing and retraining itself through neuroplasticity. When you perform repetitive physical tasks, you tap into this ability by "retraining" unaffected parts of your brain to perform functions that your damaged brain cells once performed. In simple terms, neuroplasticity is the process of "rewiring" the brain to perform tasks through different neural pathways.

Some "spontaneous" recovery does occur after a stroke, but it doesn't continue forever. According to a study published in the Journal of the American Physical Therapy Association, spontaneous motor recovery only occurs during the first 6 months of recovery. Afterwards, rehabilitation is necessary to make further progress, especially if you need to learn new skills and coping mechanisms.

"Rehabilitation involving neuroplasticity principles requires repetition of task and task-specific practice to be effective."

To overcome the leading cause of disability, a consistent exercise program is critical. By using the power of neuroplasticity, stroke survivors can regain mobility and function. If you want to overcome the limitations of traditional recovery methods, you should know that exercise is your most effective tool.

BENEFITS OF EXERCISE AFTER A STROKE

Physical activity reduces your stroke risk by between 25% and 30%, but it doesn't just decrease your risk of having a stroke. Exercise also increases your chance of regaining function after a stroke. Unfortunately, stroke survivors don't always realize that their chance of recovery may have more to do with their rehabilitation efforts than with the initial extent of their brain injury.

In fact, when stroke survivors have trouble performing daily functions, it isn't always because of the stroke itself. Brain damage also causes problems that indirectly lead to loss of physical function. After suffering a stroke, survivors who don't begin an exercise regimen will experience additional, preventable problems such as physical deconditioning and fatigue...

They may also face a variety of obstacles that make it more difficult to begin exercising, such as:

- Lack of social support
- Financial instability
- Depression
- Severity of physical symptoms
- Fatigue
- Frustration
- Confusion
- Lack of motivation

These barriers are precisely why a tailored, consistent exercise regimen is such an important part of proper post-stroke care. When patients receive support, tools, and specific instructions to keep them active after a stroke, obstacles such as fatigue and depression will get smaller and less powerful, making it easier to continue a regimen of aerobic and strength-training exercises.

These exercises, in turn, give patients the power to reclaim lost abilities and get back to the life they had before the stroke. According to the American Heart Association, exercising after a stroke is a crucial way to improve the following:

- Cardiovascular fitness
- Walking ability
- Muscle strength
- Flexibility
- Coordination
- Cognitive function
- Mental health
- Memory
- Quality of life

Any amount of physical activity is a positive step for stroke survivors. Over time, even light activity such as walking around the block or doing laundry will contribute to physical improvements and help prevent the deconditioning that leads to further deterioration. However, activities of moderate intensity are even more beneficial for your health. If you want to reclaim a specific function, for example, you can incorporate a variety of at-home exercises to target individual body parts.

EXERCISES FOR STROKE RECOVERY

Remember, a full recovery is only possible if you take direct action to reclaim function in the months and years that follow. By following an exercise program that targets specific areas and functions, you can reclaim your coordination, strength, and range of motion throughout your body.

Each of the following exercises is designed to condition your body and brain in specific ways. The movements are recommended by trusted physical therapy professionals and cover the following areas of the body: shoulders, arms, balance, hands, legs, and core. Follow along with helpful illustrations as you work through the basic, intermediate, and advanced versions of these post-stroke exercises.

RECLAIM YOUR STRENGTH WITH THESE 8 ARM EXERCISES FOR STROKE PATIENTS

A stroke can often rob a patient of arm movement, making it difficult to perform simple tasks like moving the arm forward or grasping and releasing objects. Performing basic exercises at home empowers stroke survivors to restore normal function to their arms and improve their daily lives.

Simbarashe Shahwe, the Team Lead Physiotherapist at Boston Physiotherapy Ltd. , believes in the importance of exercise in stroke recovery. After seeing numerous patients who have struggled with arm control after a stroke, Shahwe has begun encouraging patients to focus on basic arm exercises for stroke recovery in order to build strength and renew the muscle-to-mind connections often lost after a stroke.

ARM EXERCISES FOR STROKE PATIENTS

Shahwe believes that exercise is important as you focus on recovery, and also understands that the outpatient therapy may not be sufficient exercise. It often requires supplementation with at-home exercises.

As with any new exercise routine, please talk to your doctor or another qualified healthcare professional before you begin. If you have any pain or discomfort, or a worsening of your symptoms, please stop the exercises immediately.

BASIC LEVEL EXERCISES

Strokes are a frightening, life-threatening medical condition, but once you begin recovering you will experience the impact on your quality of life caused by neurological damage. It's possible to retrain the brain to make up for this damage, but you must keep the affected muscle groups active. These basic level exercises are a starting point to add flexibility and mobility to your affected arm after a stroke.

A stroke can often make it difficult to perform simple tasks like moving the arm forward or grasping and releasing objects. Physiotherapist Simbarashe Shawe recommends eight simple exercises to help restore strength and function in the arms of stroke survivors.

Exercise #1 Inner Arm Stretch

For this exercise, place your hands palms down on the table and rotate your wrist so your fingers point towards your body. Keeping your elbows straight, slowly move your body backwards until you feel a stretch on the inside of the arm. Lean on the table for support if you need to.

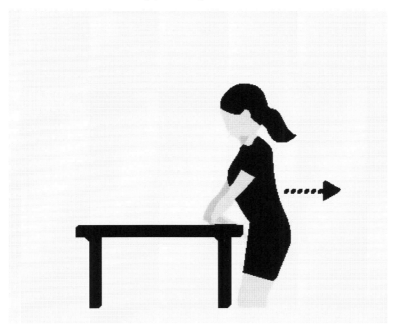

Exercise #2 Wrist and Hand Stretch

For this exercise, place your forearm on the table, with the hand over the edge of the table, palm down. First, drop the hand down, using your other hand to gently stretch the ligaments and muscles. Then, leaving your forearm on the table, lift the wrist up, down and sideways, gently stretching the extended wrist with the other hand.

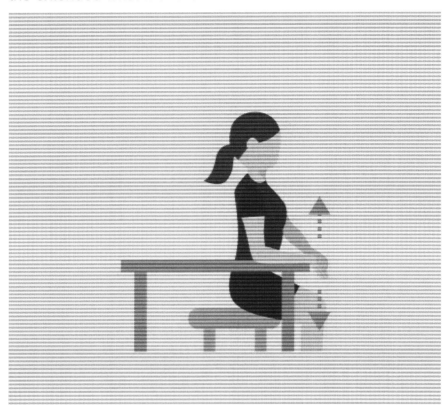

INTERMEDIATE LEVEL EXERCISE

Once you have gained basic flexibility in the wrist, hand, and inner arm, you are ready to work on a full range of motion for these joints. These intermediate-level exercises, can be the key to recovering the use of your arms. They help retrain the brain to make up for the neurological damage you have suffered.

14

Exercise #3 Elbow Stretch

The elbow stretch focuses on restoring a range of motion to the elbow. This exercise can be done while sitting or standing. Hold the arm at a comfortable position, then carefully bend and straighten the elbows as if you are doing a dumbbell curl.

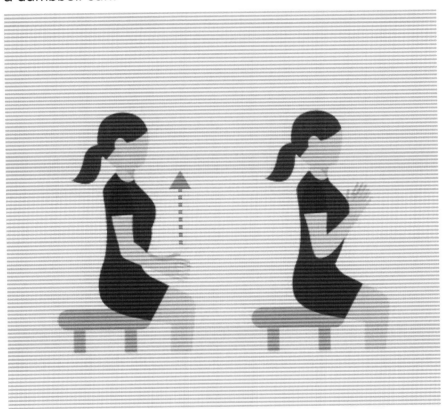

Exercise #4 Crawling Stretch

Take up a crawling position with your elbows straight. Gently lean your body backwards, keeping your arm position, until you feel a stretch on your inner arm. Hold the position and repeat.

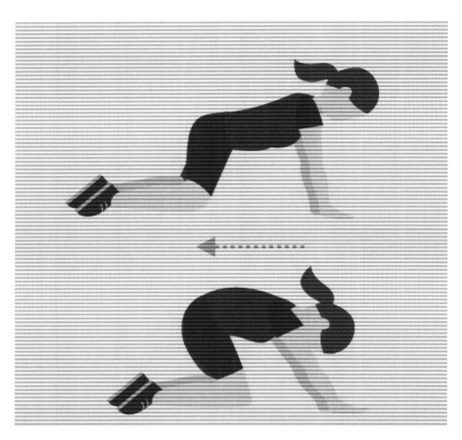

Exercise #5 Wrist Motion

When you are sitting or standing, extend the elbow and rotate your wrist through a full range of motion. Continue this exercise a few times to encourage greater motion in the wrist.

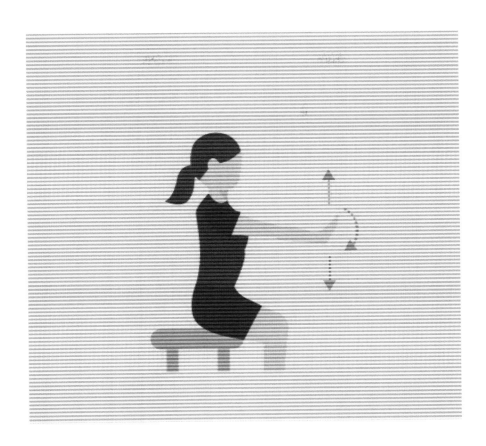

ADVANCED LEVEL EXERCISE

Muscles damaged due to a stroke are often weakened, mainly due to inactivity. This is why at-home exercise is so important. Once you have regained range of motion in your arm and wrist, you are ready to begin strengthening the muscles with these advanced exercises.

Exercise #6 Elbow Weight Training

In a standing or sitting position, hold a small weight in your hand. Gently bend and straighten the elbow. Repeat to your endurance point. Over time, increase repetitions as the elbow strengthens.

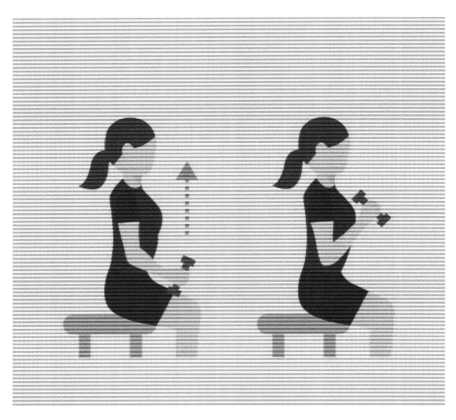

Exercise #7 Finger Walk

Stand facing a wall or a door. Place your fingers gently on the surface of the door or wall. Walk your fingers up the surface using a spider-like motion, then walk them back down.

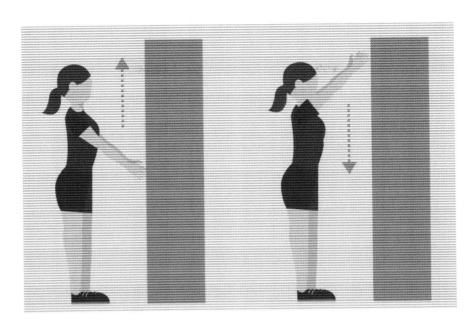

Exercise #8 Seated Pushup

Finally, sit on the ground with your knees bent and your palms on the floor, keeping your fingers pointing forward. Push through your hands to cause your bottom to lift off the floor slightly. Repeat as you grow stronger.

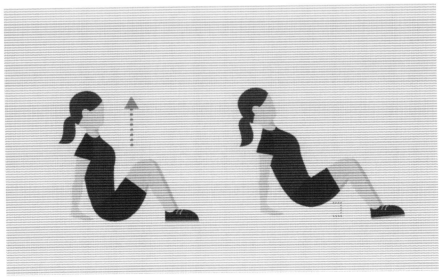

THE IMPORTANCE OF ARM EXERCISE FOR FULL STROKE RECOVERY

Stroke is a common problem for people after the age of 65, and your risk increases after the age of 55. The CDC estimates that nearly 800,000 people in the United States will suffer from a stroke each year, causing one person to die every four minutes. Those who do survive may suffer a poor quality of life due to the effects of neurological damage. A stroke is a serious medical condition with far-reaching consequences.

Stroke survivors do not have to assume that the struggles they have are permanent. Quality of life can be preserved with a proactive approach to stroke recovery. These arm exercises for stroke recovery can be some of the most effective techniques to improve arm range of motion and strength. If you have lost mobility in your arms due to a stroke, you can take back control and put recovery in your own hands with the help of simple arm exercises.

RECLAIM YOUR STABILITY WITH THESE BALANCE EXERCISES FOR STROKE RECOVERY

If you are struggling to walk or are stumbling often after a stroke, the problem may be muscle weakness, but it could also be your balance. A stroke damages the brain and weakens the messages your ears, eyes and muscles sent to the neurological system. These messages are essential to maintaining balance. As the brain begins to repair itself, you may notice a return of your coordination and balance. However, residual balance problems may occur, especially if the stroke affected your vision, hearing, or the balance control system in the brain.

For patients who are not seeing improvement in balance in the first several months of recovery, physical and occupational therapy can help restore that balance. However, balance is an ability that has to be relearned after a stroke, and that requires more attention than physical therapy alone can provide. In addition to physical therapy in a clinic, at-home balance exercises for stroke recovery can help restore balance again.

BALANCE EXERCISES FOR STROKE RECOVERY

Beth Thornton and Kathryn Smyth, two physiotherapists at Physio at Home, recommend a system of at-home exercises to help patients restore their balance as they regain this crucial skill. They believe that giving patients the skills to do these exercises at home will help improve their chances of healing.

While these exercises represent minimal risk, you should always discuss your plans with a doctor before beginning a new exercise program. Do not continue exercising if you experience pain or discomfort, but talk to your doctor right away.

BASIC LEVEL BALANCE EXERCISES

Basic level exercises for balance may seem simple at first, but they require strong neural connections to successfully complete. Start with these simple exercises as you work to rewire your mental processes. The repeated actions will build mental connections that can help restore balance. Remember, for these basic level exercises, always hold onto something to ensure you do not fall.

Exercise 1: Heel Raises (Holding On)

3 sets of 10

Find a sturdy chair or countertop you can hold onto for support. Hold onto the chair or counter, and raise yourself up onto your tiptoes, keeping your knees straight and holding your upper body tall. Lower yourself back to the floor slowly, and repeat.

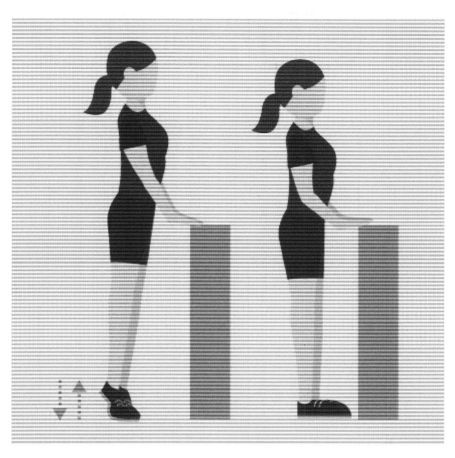

Exercise 2: Side Stepping (Holding On)

3 sets of 10 (1 rep = both feet)

Use a counter or ledge to hold on to, or ask someone to give you a hand to hold for balance. Place tape on the floor in a straight line. Step sideways to cross the line, crossing one leg across the front of the other leg. Reverse the motion to return to the starting point, this time crossing a leg behind.

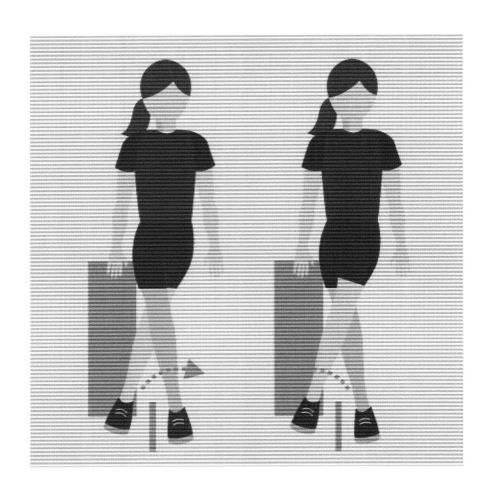

INTERMEDIATE LEVEL BALANCE EXERCISES

The intermediate level exercises use the same basic ideas as the basic exercises, but without something to hold onto. After practicing the basic level exercises for a while, you should be able to perform them without assistance. However, for safety, always have a counter or chair nearby to grab if you start to lose your balance.

Exercise 3: Heel Raises (Not Holding On)

3 sets of 10

Stand with your feet flat on the floor and your arms at your sides. Raise yourself to tiptoe, keeping your upper body and knees straight. Slowly lower and repeat.

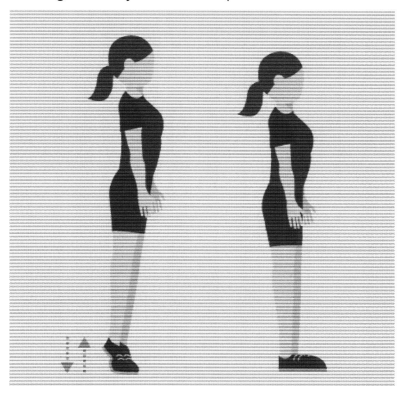

Exercise 4: Side Stepping (Not Holding On)

3 sets of 10 (1 rep = both feet)

Perform the side step, crossing your legs across each other as you move sideways across a straight line, but without holding on. Go slowly to avoid a fall, and be ready to grab a hold of something if you lose your balance.

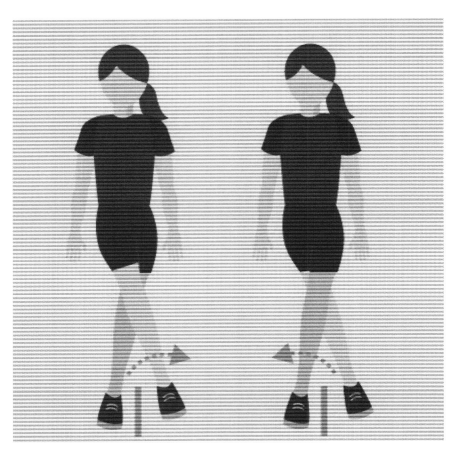

Exercise 5: Heel-to-Toe Walking

20 steps (10 for each foot)

Using the straight tape line for side stepping, walk forward, placing the heel of your foot directly in front of the toe of your other foot as you walk. Continue to the end of the tape, turn, and repeat by returning to the starting point.

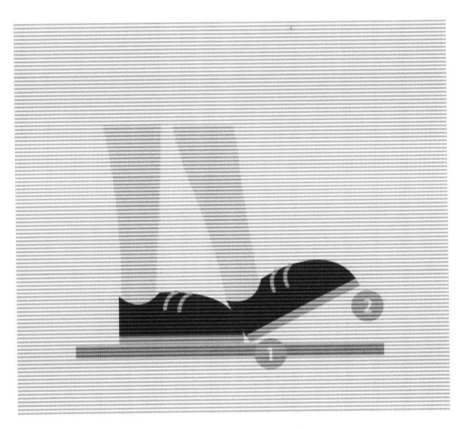

Exercise 6: Squats Against Gym Ball

3 sets of 10

Place an exercise ball between your back and a wall, standing tall. Slowly lower into a squatting position, holding on with one hand if needed or not holding on at all. Roll back up to a standing position and repeat.

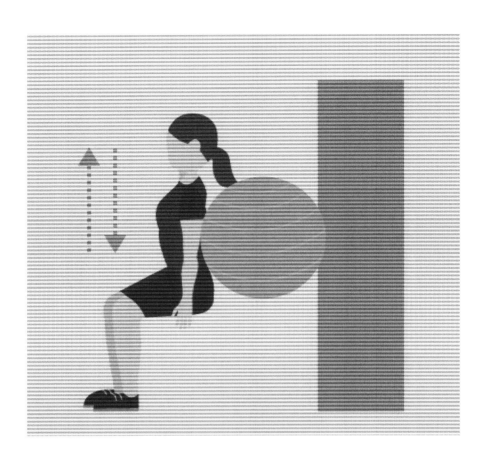

ADVANCED LEVEL BALANCE EXERCISES

Once you start noticing improved balance, do not stop exercising. You are still building those connections. Now it's time to move on to advanced level exercises.

Exercise 7: Single Leg Standing

3 sets of 5

Place both feet flat on the floor. Slowly lift one leg until you are balanced on the other leg. Hold for a count of 10, and slowly lower it back down. Alternate legs and repeat.

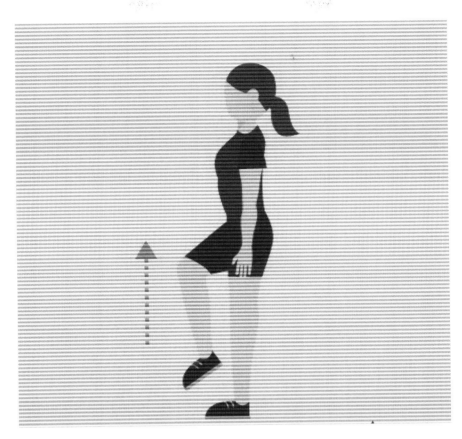

Exercise 8: Backwards Walking

20 steps

In a room that is free from obstacles, walk backwards slowly. Try to avoid looking where you are going, but use your sense of balance and slow movements to avoid a fall. At first, perform this exercise with something closeby to hold onto like a wall or countertop until you gain confidence in your abilities.

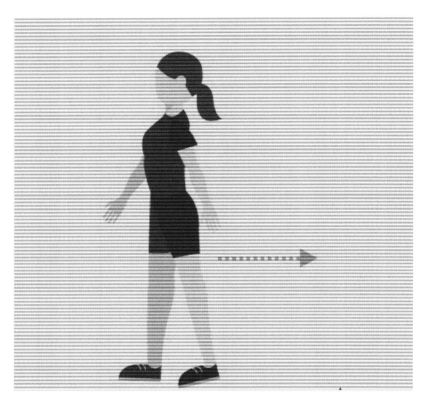

Exercise 9: Weighted Ball Pass

3 sets of 10

Using a weighted exercise ball, slowly pass the ball from hand to hand as you circle it around your body. Start by circling the body in a clockwise motion. Then, repeat in a counter-clockwise motion. Perform this exercise while standing.

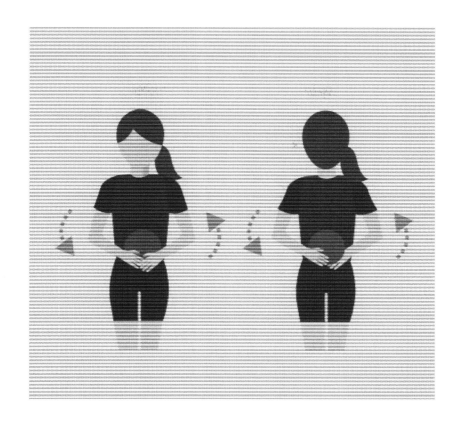

FINDING BALANCE AGAIN WILL IMPROVE MANY ASPECTS OF LIFE AFTER STROKE

In the United States alone, 600,000 people will suffer from a stroke every single year, and as many as 30 percent of those patients will have ongoing physical problems as a result. For some, that will include a loss of balance. Losing your sense of balance changes many aspects of life. Simple actions, like rising out of a chair, become increasingly complex and require a tremendous amount of thought and effort. With a careful exercise routine at home like these balance exercises for stroke recovery, combined with physical and occupational therapy, you can limit these problems and enjoy a full life, even after a serious stroke.

RECLAIM YOUR STABILITY WITH CORE EXERCISES FOR STROKE RECOVERY

While the focus of stroke recovery is often on the limbs and facial muscles, without a strong core, the rest of the body may suffer. By isolating and activating core muscles with nine exercises selected by Thornton and Smyth, stroke survivors can work to regain coordination and strength that benefits their whole body.

As with any new exercise, stroke victims should talk with their healthcare provider before attempting any of these. If the exercises cause pain, the individual should stop.

BASIC LEVEL CORE STRENGTH EXERCISES

Strokes are life-threatening events that can cause irreversible neurological damage, so the recovery period is as much about retraining the brain as it is about strengthening the muscles. In order to regain use of your core muscles, you must keep them active in order to create the brain connections you need to improve after a stroke.

When first starting out, consider practicing these basic level core exercises:

1) PELVIC FLOOR CONTRACTIONS

Pelvic floor contractions, also known as Kegels, can help strengthen the muscles on the pelvic floor, which is the muscular base of the abdomen attached to the pelvis.

First, find the muscles by imagining that you are trying to hold urine or stop from passing gas. Squeeze these muscles by lifting and drawing in, then hold for a count of three. Relax then repeat, gradually increasing the holding time until you can hold for 10 seconds.

If at any point you feel the contraction relaxing, let it relax completely and rest for 10 seconds before contracting again. Repeat the exercise 10 times.

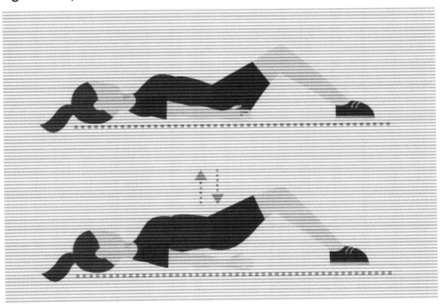

2) KNEE ROLLING

Lay on your back with your hands resting at your side. Bend your knees and place your feet flat on the floor. Roll your hips so that your knees push to the left, then to the right, then back to center. Repeat 10-20 times.

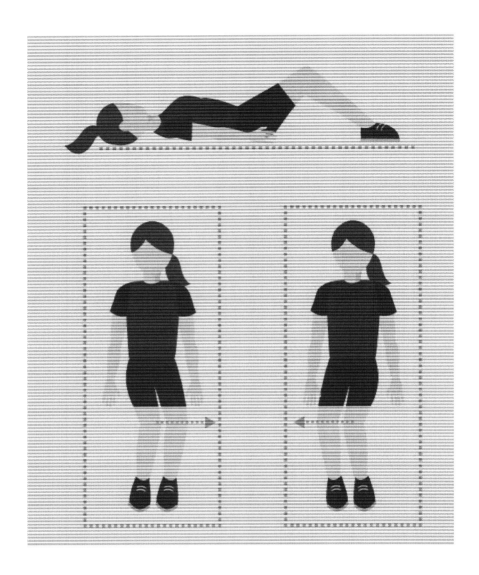

3) SINGLE LEG DROP-OUTS

Lay on the floor with the hips and feet flat with the knees bent. Keep the pelvis still, using the hands to keep it in place if needed. Inhale, and drop the left knee to the left, as far as possible without lifting the pelvis, keeping the knee bent. Exhale, and draw the knee back in. Repeat 5 times per side.

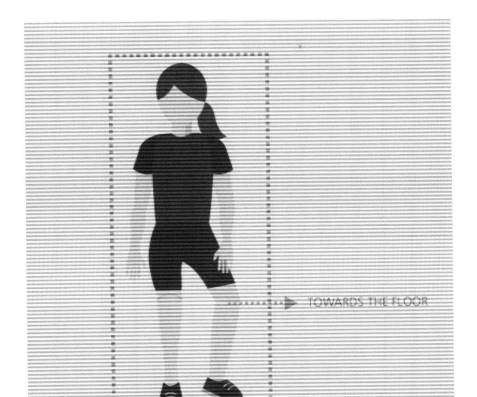

TOWARDS THE FLOOR

INTERMEDIATE LEVEL CORE STRENGTH EXERCISES

Once you begin building some strength, you are ready to progress in your exercise practice. These intermediate exercises will challenge a larger number of core muscles and build even more strength.

4) SINGLE LEG BRIDGING

Lay on the exercise mat and place one leg flat on the floor with the knee bent. Place the other leg on an exercise ball. Using the core muscles, lift the pelvis off the mat and slowly lower back down. Repeat for 10 repetitions, then switch legs.

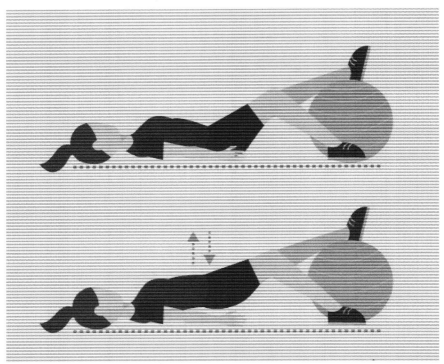

5) SIDE LAYING CLAMS

Clams are a great exercise for your core as well as your legs. Lie down on your side with your knees bent, resting one knee on top of the other. Keeping your feet together, lift the upper knee towards the ceiling and hold your knees apart for 10 seconds. Next, slowly lower your knee back down. Be careful not to roll your hips back. Repeat 5-10 times on each side.

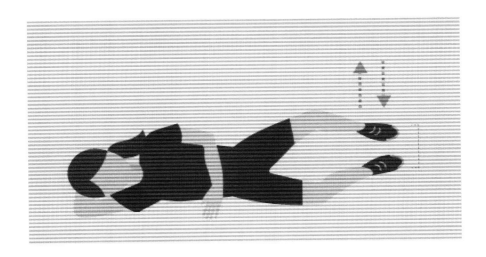

6) FOUR-POINT KNEELING

Kneel on the ground and place your hands flat on the ground so you are in a crawling stance. Contract the pelvic floor and raise one leg while lifting the opposite arm. Hold for a few seconds, and return to the starting position, repeating with the opposite arm and leg. Repeat for two to three sets of 10 reps each.

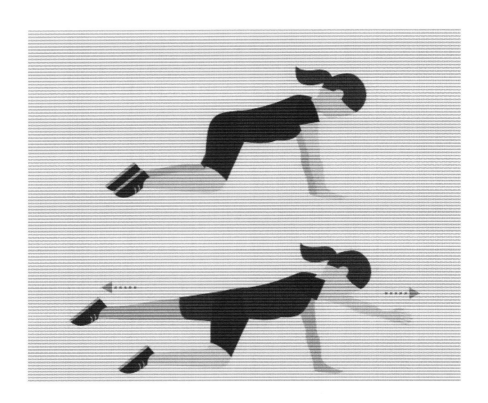

ADVANCED LEVEL EXERCISES

As you continue to develop your core muscles, you will be ready to add more intensity. These advanced exercises increase the intensity of the intermediate exercises so you can regain a strong, healthy core.

7) BRIDGING WITH ARMS ABOVE HEAD

Lay on an exercise mat with your shoulders and lower back flat on the floor. Support your legs on an exercise ball. Lift your arms above your head, then use the core muscles to lift your hips off the floor until your body is in a straight line from heels to shoulders. Slowly lower back down and repeat 10-15 times.

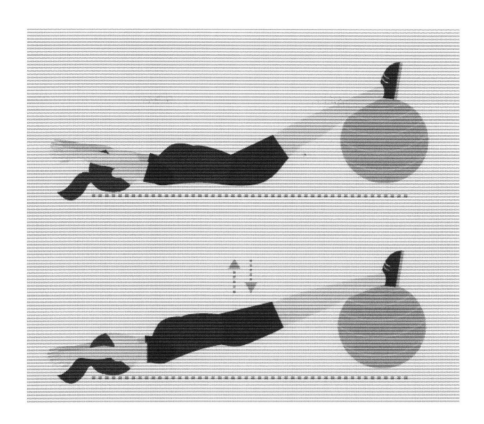

8) BILATERAL LEG CYCLING

Lay on the floor and lift the legs off of the ground, holding them in a cycling position. Then, cycle as if you are riding a bicycle in the air. Rest and repeat 10 times.

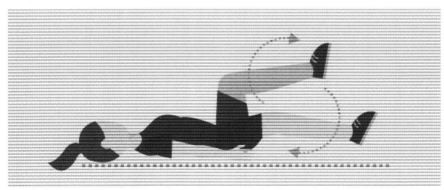

39

9) SUPERMAN POSE

Imagine superman flying through the air. Now, lay on the floor on your stomach and take this same position, arms and legs extended. Hold to strengthen the core muscles in your back, and relax. Hold the position for 2-5 seconds and repeat 10 times.

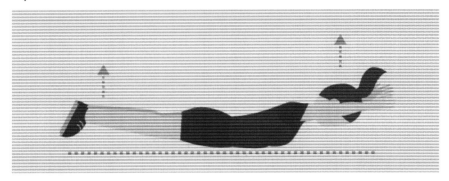

WHEN RETRAINING THE BRAIN AND BODY AFTER A STROKE, DON'T NEGLECT THE CORE

A stroke is a life-altering event that can happen in an instance. For many stroke patients, it serves as a wake up call to pay closer attention to health and wellness. A pro-active approach to retraining the muscles and the brain after a stroke is a great first step towards a healthier life.

When working at home, do not neglect those crucial core muscles. With a little bit of attention to the core, and the help of products to strengthen the hands, arms, and shoulders, you can experience a high quality of life after a stroke.

RECLAIM YOUR DEXTERITY WITH 25 HAND EXERCISES FOR STROKE RECOVERY

When stroke survivors lose function and dexterity in the hands, simple daily tasks can seem like insurmountable obstacles. Sarah Lyon, occupational therapist, advocates three simple, at-home exercises to help stroke survivors regain the use of their hands.

A stroke can take a seemingly healthy and vibrant individual and change their life in an instant. Learning how to do basic daily tasks, such as self-feeding or getting dressed each day, can quickly feel like an overwhelming physical hurdle. Despite having full active movement in your affected hand, you may have decreased strength and dexterity in your hand due to your stroke. This may be making it difficult to grasp and release objects, making daily tasks seem like insurmountable obstacles. We will show you some helpful hand exercises for stroke recovery to help you reclaim your strength and dexterity.

Unfortunately, sometimes rehab does not bring back full control and use of your hands, making these daily tasks a tremendous challenge. While you begin your recovery it's crucial that you incorporate hand exercises for stroke recovery into your daily life to bring back dexterity and use of your   fingers.

THERAPEUTIC BALL EXERCISES FOR HAND RECOVERY AFTER STROKE

Therapeutic balls are extremely useful for building strength and dexterity, especially in the aftermath of a stroke event. They are widely available, in a range of resistance levels, and affordable.

EXERCISE #1: BALL GRIP

Hold ball tightly in palm of hand. Squeeze the ball, hold, and relax. Repeat ten times, for two sets.

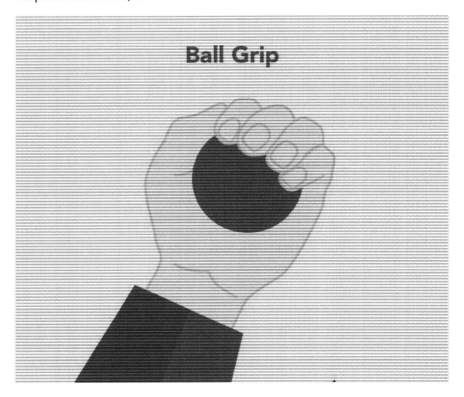

Ball Grip

EXERCISE #2: THUMB EXTEND

Place ball between bent thumb and extended two fingers of same hand. Extend and straighten the thumb to roll the ball. Repeat ten times, for two sets.

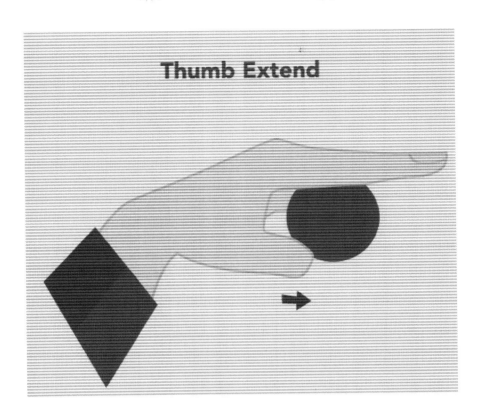

Thumb Extend

EXERCISE #3: PINCH

Hold ball between thumb and index and middlefingers. Squeeze together, hold and relax. Repeat ten times, for two sets.

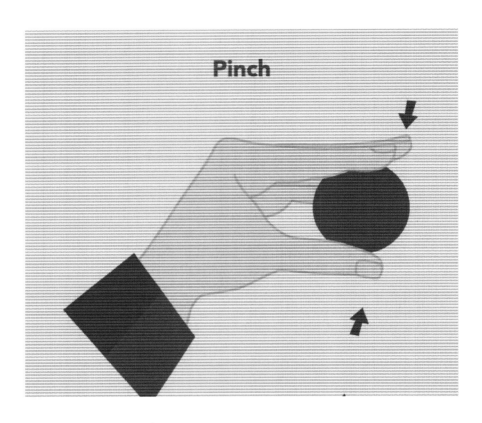

EXERCISE #4: OPPOSITION

Place ball in palm of hand, bringing thumb towards the base of the little finger.Repeat ten times, for two sets.

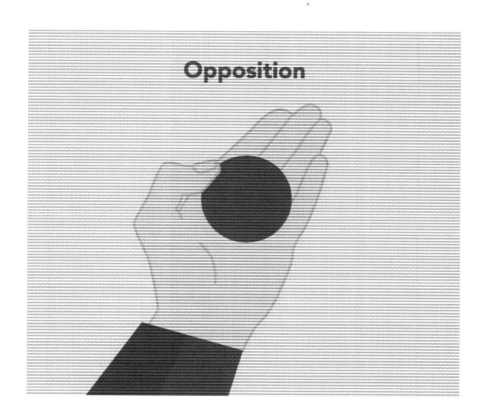

Opposition

EXERCISE #5: SIDE SQUEEZE

Place ball between any two fingers. Squeeze the two fingers together, hold and relax. Repeat ten times, for two sets.

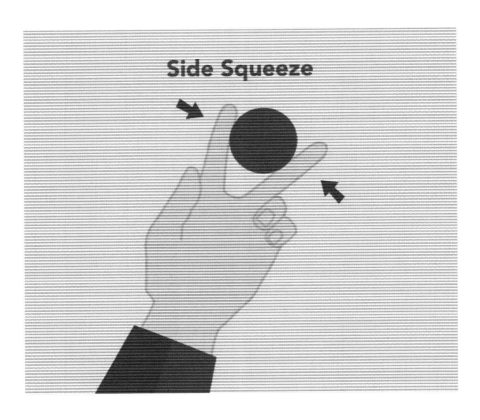

Side Squeeze

EXERCISE #6: EXTEND OUT

Place ball on a table. Place tips of fingers on the ball and roll the ball outward on the table. Repeat ten times, for two sets.

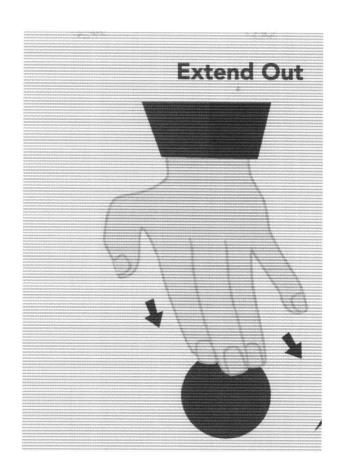

THERAPEUTIC PUTTY EXERCISES FOR HAND RECOVERY AFTER STROKE

Therapeutic putty is an extremely useful tool for building strength and dexterity, especially in the aftermath of a stroke event. It is widely available, in a variety of resistance levels, and affordable.

EXERCISE #7: SCISSOR SPREAD

Wrap putty around two fingers and try to spread the fingers apart. Repeat ten times, for two sets.

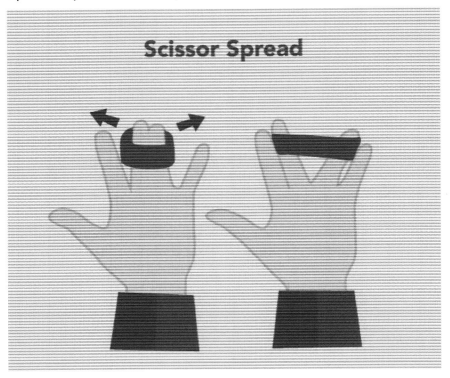

Scissor Spread

EXERCISE #8: THUMB PRESS

Place putty in palm of hand and push into it with the thumb towards the base ofthe small finger. Repeat ten times, for two sets.

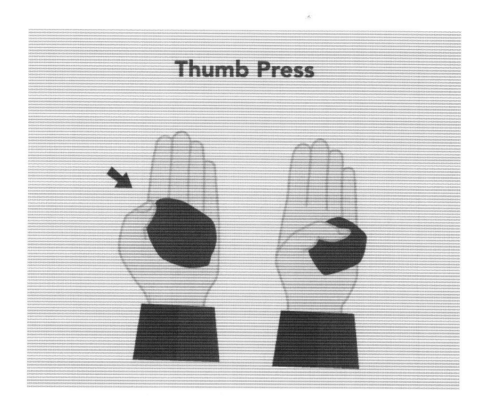
Thumb Press

EXERCISE #9: THUMB EXTENSION

Bend thumb and loop clay around it. Try to straighten thumb as if simulating a "thumbs up" gesture. Repeat ten times, for two sets.

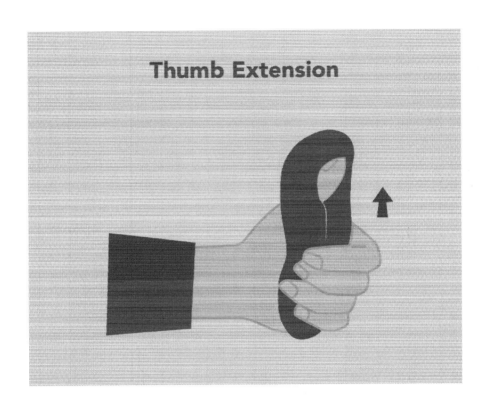

EXERCISE #10: THUMB PINCH STRENGTHENING

Squeeze puttybetween thumb and side of index finger. Repeat ten times, for two sets.

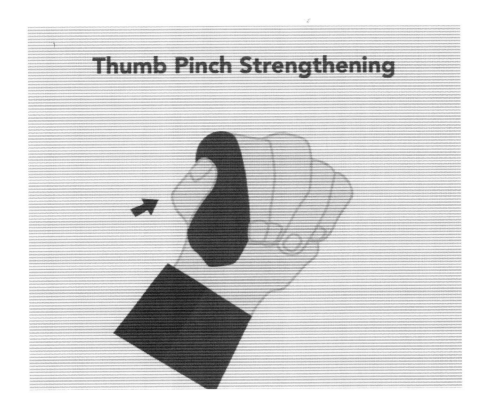

Thumb Pinch Strengthening

EXERCISE #11: THUMB ADDUCTION

Keep fingers and thumb straight while pressing the putty between index finger and thumb. Repeat ten times, for two sets.

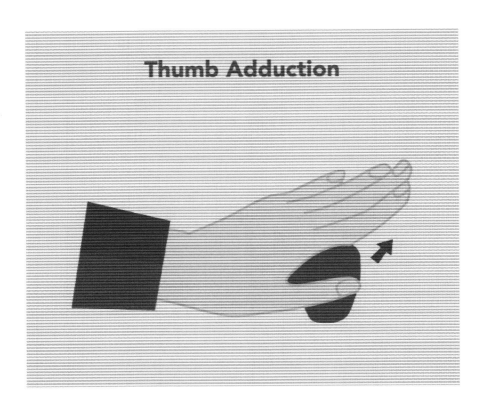

Thumb Adduction

EXERCISE #12: THREE JAW CHUCK PINCH

Using thumb, index and middle finger, pull putty upwards.
Repeat ten times, for two sets.

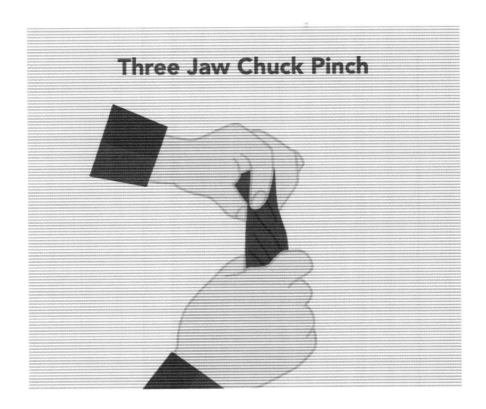

Three Jaw Chuck Pinch

EXERCISE #13: FINGER HOOK

Place putty in palm of hand and press fingers into a hook shape, attempting to only bend the two last joints of the fingers. Repeat ten times, for two sets.

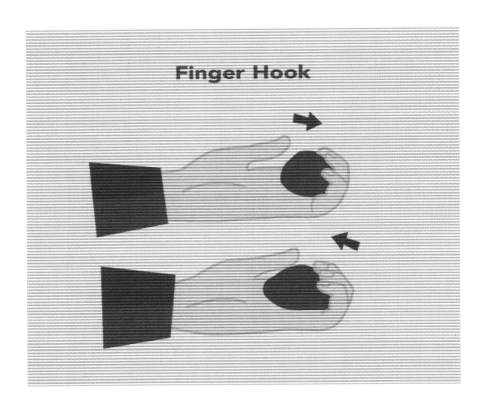

EXERCISE #14: FULL GRIP

Place putty in palm of hand and make a fist while squeezing fingers into the clay. Repeat ten times, for two sets.

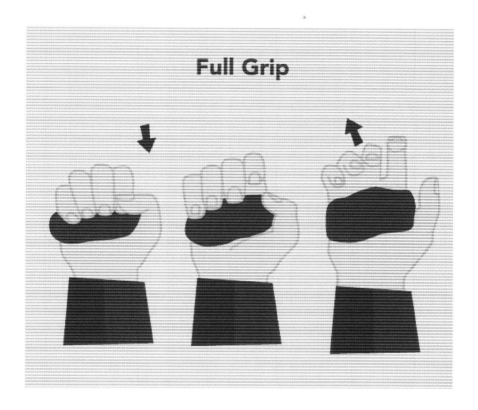

Full Grip

EXERCISE #15: FINGER PINCH

Pinch the putty between each finger and the thumb. Repeat ten times for each finger, for two sets.

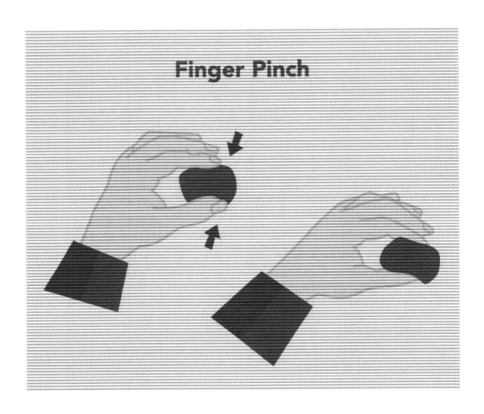

Finger Pinch

EXERCISE #16: FINGER EXTENSION

Bend finger and loop putty around it. Try to straighten finger. Repeat ten times, to each finger for two sets.

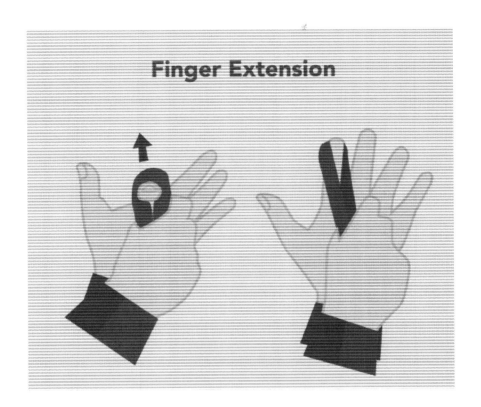

Finger Extension

EXERCISE #17: FINGER SCISSOR

Take a 1" diameter ball of putty and place between fingers. Squeeze and release. Repeat ten times, for each finger for two sets.

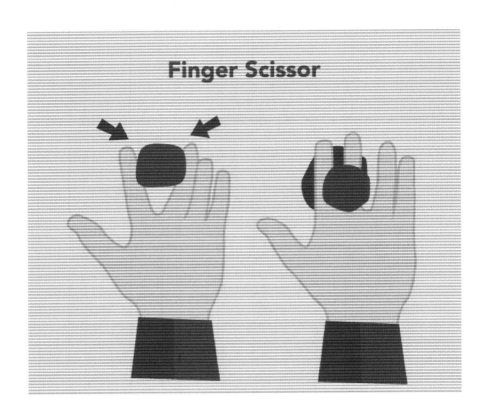

EXERCISE #18: FINGER SPREAD

Spread a pancake of putty over the fingers. Try to spread them apart. Repeat ten times, for two sets.

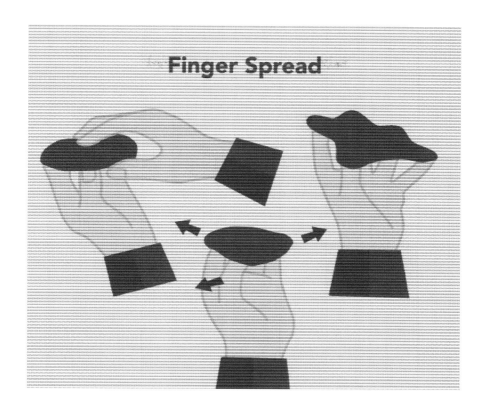

HAND RECOVERY EXERCISES WITH EVERYDAY HOUSEHOLD ITEMS

It is possible that a survivor will not have therapeutic putty or a ball handy when they would like to exercise their hand. Fortunately, there are many exercises one can perform using just their body or common objects like coins or water bottles.

EXERCISE #19: ROLL MOVEMENT

Place the affected arm on the table and place a water bottle in the affected hand. Keep the affected hand and fingers relaxed. Curl the fingers in and grasp the water bottle then release. Repeat ten times, for two sets.

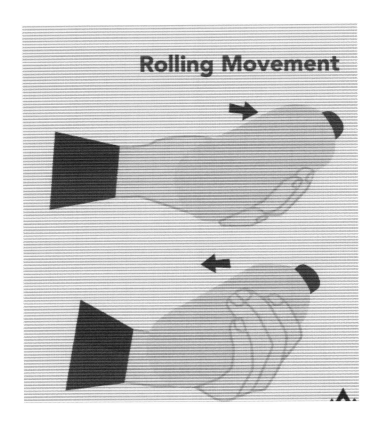

Rolling Movement

EXERCISE #20: WRIST CURL

Grasp the water bottle in the affected hand and use the non-affected hand to prop and support the affected arm. Allow the wrist to stretch down, and then curl the wrist up. Repeat ten times, for two sets.

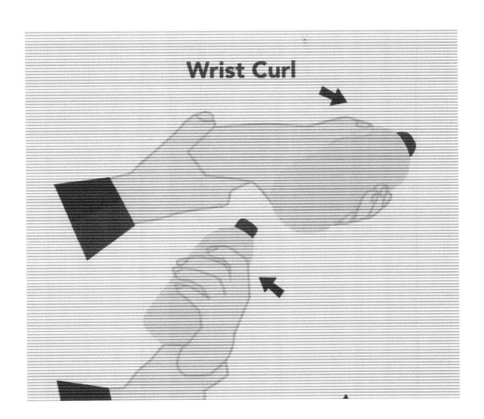

EXERCISE #21: WRIST EXTEND

Grasp the water bottle in the affected hand and use the non-affected hand to prop and support the affected arm. Position the hand so the palm is facing down, then extend the wrist. Repeat ten times, for two sets.

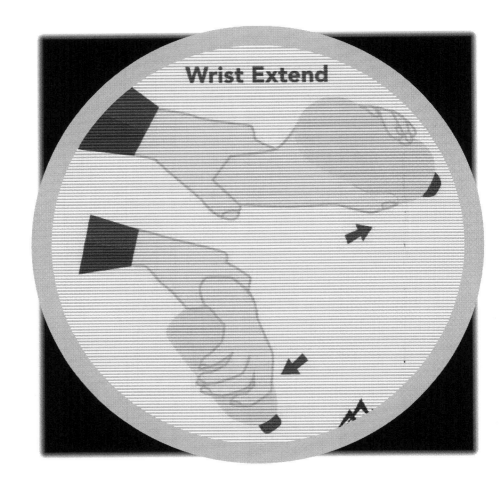

EXERCISE #22: PINCH & RELEASE

Place a pen to the side of the table and then gently grip it with the affected fingers. Slide the pen across the table, and then release. Repeat ten times, for two sets.

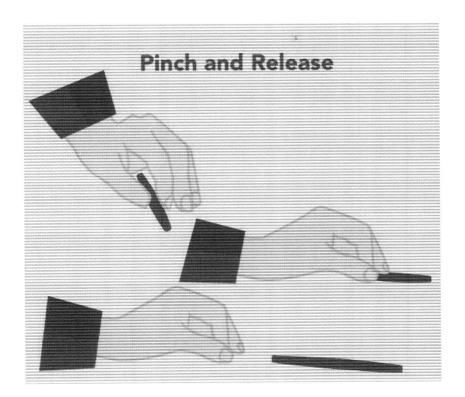

Pinch and Release

EXERCISE #23: PEN SPIN

Place a pen on the table and use the thumb and fingers to spin it. Try not to involve the shoulder in this exercise: the objective is to isolate the thumb and fingers. Aim for speed during this exercise, if possible, by spinning the pen quickly for 15 seconds.

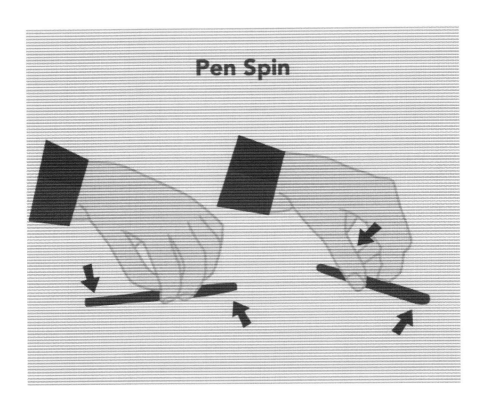

Pen Spin

EXERCISE #24: COIN DROP

Place 8 quarters in a row in the palm of the affected hand. Then, use the thumb to slide one quarter down into the index finger and thumb. Pinch the quarter with your index finger and thumb. Then, place the quarter down onto the table while keeping the other quarters in \hand using the other fingers. Repeat with the remaining quarters.

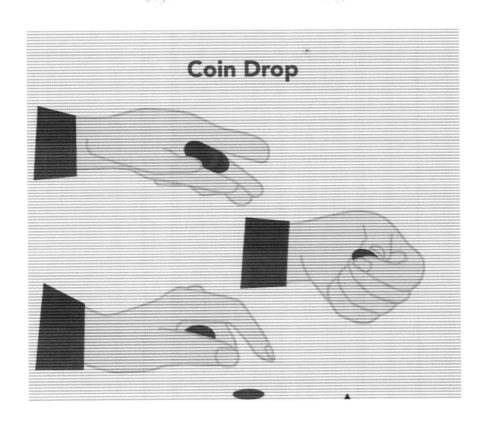

EXERCISE #25: FINGER OPPOSITION

Bend the affected arm, placing the elbow on the table. Bring the tip of the index finger to the tip of the thumb to make a ring. Pinch, and release. Repeat with your middle, ring, and pinkie finger. Pinch, and release. Perform with each finger, for two sets.

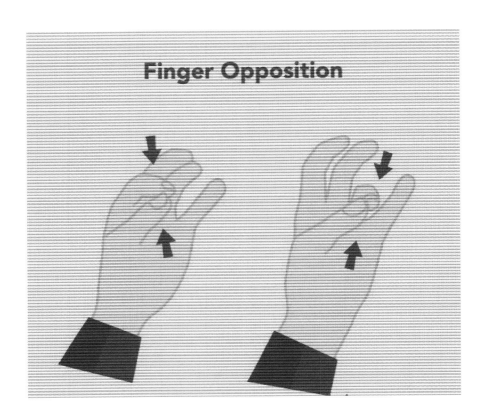

STROKE RECOVERY HAND AND FINGER EXERCISES CAN IMPROVE QUALITY OF LIFE

The ability to use your hands to grasp and release objects, type at a computer, button a shirt, or even write a note to someone you love is so important to a high quality of life. If your stroke has robbed you of this ability, take action to improve your quality of life by beginning an at-home exercise program. These finger and hand exercises for stroke recovery can help you regain the use and dexterity in your hands as you retrain your brain after the neurological damage that was caused from your stroke.

RECLAIM MOBILITY WITH LEG EXERCISES FOR STROKE RECOVERY

Difficulties standing and walking after a stroke can be related to balance problems, but leg strength and mobility are also contributing factors. Richard Sealy recommends a series of low-impact strength and stretching exercises to help regain muscle in the legs and improve range of motion during stroke recovery.

Stroke recovery can be a long process. Managing the ongoing need to rebuild bodily control and strength after neurological damage is no easy task. Each year nearly 800,000 people in the United States alone will suffer from a stroke, leaving them with ongoing physical and neurological damage.

If you have suffered from a stroke, loss of balance and control can make standing and walking difficult. While outpatient stroke recovery therapy is vital to improving this problem, you can also continue improving after returning home with the help of these leg exercises for stroke recovery.

LEG EXERCISES FOR STROKE RECOVERY

Richard Sealy, director of The Rehab Practice, a private neuro-therapy rehabilitation program in the United Kingdom, regularly works with individuals, families, and caregivers to establish custom exercise routines to aid in recovery from from long-term neurological problems, like the damage caused by stroke. While he acknowledges that each patient should have a custom exercise routine specific and personal to their struggles, he recommends a series of exercises to help strengthen the legs and improve range of motion during stroke recovery.

Sealy understands the importance of fast progress after a stroke, and including ongoing at-home exercises can improve health and well-being.

As with any exercise program, please consult your healthcare provider before you begin. If you notice increased pain, discomfort, or other troubling systems, stop these exercises immediately and talk to your doctor.

EXERCISE SET 1: STANDING AND BALANCE

Balance and coordination are often lost after a stroke. This can make simple actions, like standing and walking, difficult. In addition, weakness can occur around the muscles on the exterior of the hip area.

Exercises for standing and balance are vital to helping you regain your quality of life after a stroke. When performing these exercises, always hold onto a table or similar stable surface to avoid a fall.

EXERCISE 1: BASIC LEVEL STANDING AND BALANCE EXERCISE: ASSISTED LATERAL LEG SWINGS

Hold on to a stable surface, standing straight and tall while you transfer your weight to one side. Swing the other leg to the side. Use your balance to hold this position for 10 seconds. Slowly lower your leg back down. Repeat a few times, as long as you have the strength, and then switch legs.

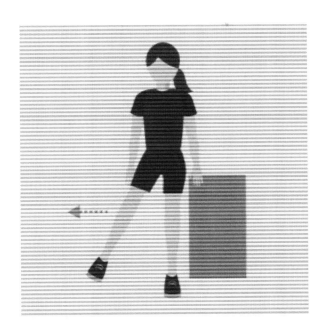

EXERCISE 2: INTERMEDIATE STANDING AND BALANCE EXERCISES: ASSISTED KNEE RAISES

Once you have mastered the first exercise, move on to the intermediate level. Again, hold on to a stable surface, keeping your back tall and straight. Transfer your weight to one leg, and bring the other leg up in front of you, bending the knee. Hold this position for a count of 10, and slowly lower it back down. Repeat, then switch legs.

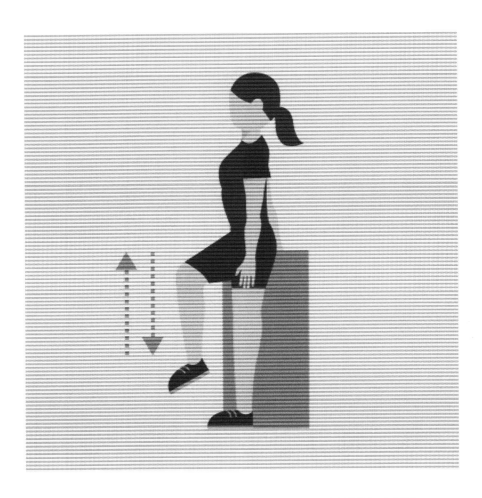

EXERCISE 3: ADVANCED STANDING AND BALANCE EXERCISES: ASSISTED REVERSE LEG SWINGS

Finally, progress to the advanced level. This time, stand straight and tall and transfer your weight to one leg. Swing the other leg out behind you as far as you can. Hold for 10 seconds, if you can, and lower it back down slowly. Repeat and switch legs.

This progression of exercises will strengthen the hip muscle and improve balance, so you can regain normal use of your legs.

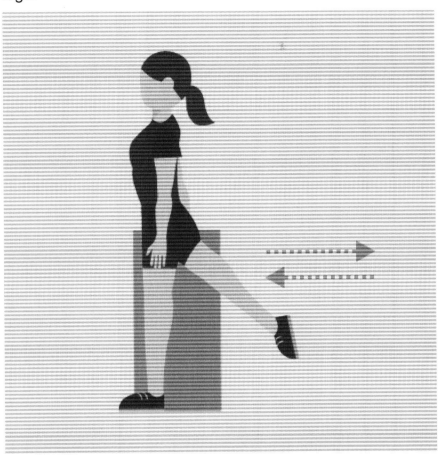

EXERCISE SET 2: BRIDGING

Often after a stroke, the hips and the core muscle groups, which are crucial to standing and walking, become weak. Bridging exercises help to strengthen these core muscles. Like the standing and balance exercises, bridging exercises move through a progression to help rebuild your strength and coordination.

EXERCISE 4: BASIC BRIDGING EXERCISE – "INNER RANGE QUAD MOVEMENT" LEG RAISES

The basic bridging exercise, called "Inner Range Quad Movement", builds strength in the thigh muscles. To perform this exercise, lay down and place a pillow or rolled towel under the knee joint. Then, press the back of the knee into the pillow or rolled towel to lift your heel off the floor.

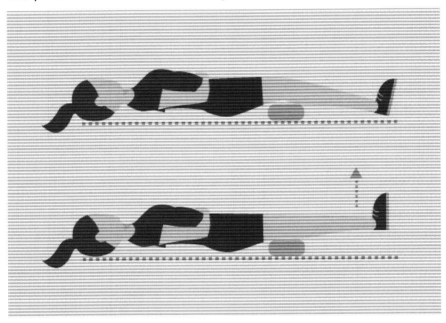

EXERCISE 5: INTERMEDIATE BRIDGING EXERCISE: SKI SQUATS – WALL SITS

"Ski Squats" take bridging exercises to the next level. For this exercise, lean against a flat wall, placing your feet in front of you. Using the wall to support your weight and your back, slowly bend your knees to lower yourself down. Hold this position for 10 seconds, if you can. Slide back up, supporting your weight on the wall, until you are in a standing position.

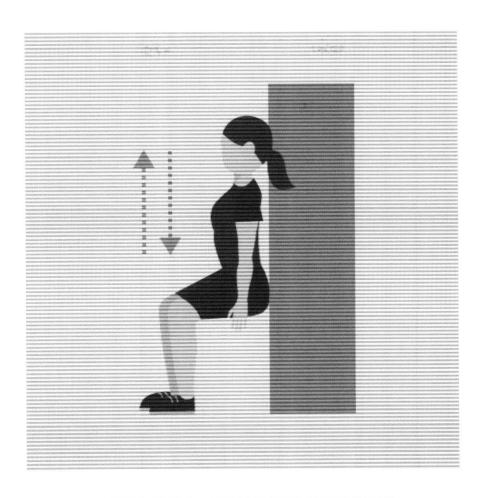

EXERCISE 6: ADVANCED BRIDGING EXERCISE SKI SQUATS – WALL SITS WITH PILATES BALL

To take bridging exercises to the advanced level, repeat the "Ski Squat", but place a gym ball between yourself and the wall when you bend your knees into the squat position.

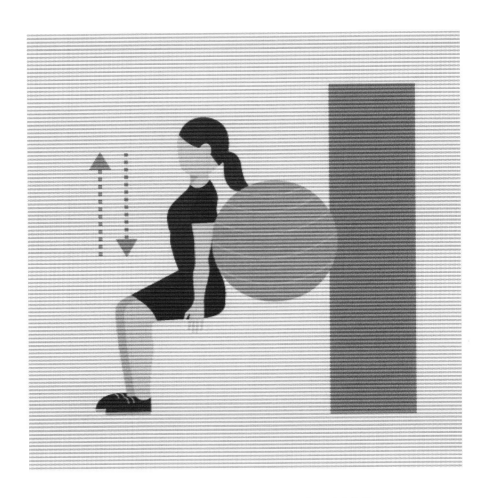

EXERCISE SET 3: CLAMS

If the lower legs are affected after a stroke, Clams can provide strengthening and improved range of motion. Clams focuses on building strength and coordination in the lower leg, increasing range of motion and control.

EXERCISE 7: BASIC CLAMS EXERCISE – IN SITTING

Before starting Clams, you must stretch the calf muscle and build coordination in the lower body. In Sitting helps with this. In a sitting position, create a stirrup around one foot using a towel or belt, placing the stirrup around the ball of the foot. Gently pull the stirrup up towards your body to stretch the calf muscle. Then, pull it with the outer hand to turn the foot out, continuing to stretch the muscle.

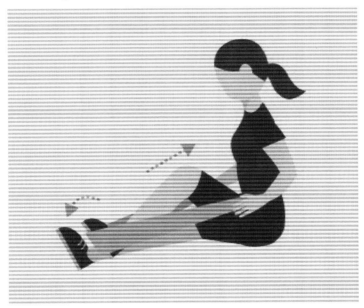

EXERCISE 8: INTERMEDIATE CLAMS EXERCISE – HIP OPENERS

Once you have build some flexibility, you are ready for the Clams exercise. Lay down on your side, and bend your knees, resting one on top of the other. Then, while you keep your feet together, lift the upper knee away from the other knee, holding them apart for a count of 10 seconds. Slowly lower your knee back down. While performing this exercise, make sure that you do not roll your hips back.

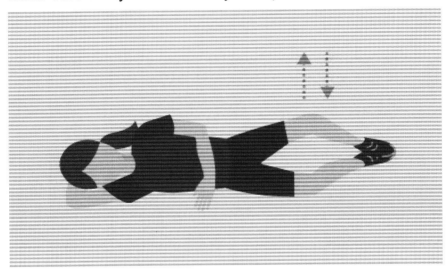

EXERCISE 9: ADVANCED CLAMS EXERCISE

After mastering Clams, take it to the next level by lifting the knee and the foot of the upper leg. Again, hold the position for a count of 10 seconds. Lower it back down. Repeat a few times to build strength and range of motion.

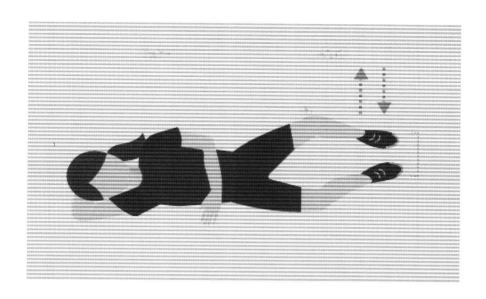

REBUILD STRENGTH AND COORDINATION WITH STROKE RECOVERY EXERCISES

Strokes can occur in people of any age, although nearly 75% of all strokes occur after the age of 65, and an individual's risk doubles after 55. Each year, approximately 600,000 people suffer from their first stroke, and an additional 185,000 have a recurrent stroke.

If you have suffered one or more strokes, it can be easy to feel discouraged at the lack of mobility and control you experience. Stroke exercises, like these, can help you regain that control and build up your strength again, so you can recover from the neurological damage of a stroke.

Many daily movements depend on shoulder strength such as grasping and releasing objects, moving the arms, and supporting weight with the arms. Occupational therapist Hoang Tran recommends six effective techniques based on the principles of gravity compensation to speed up recovery in the shoulders after a stroke.

RECLAIM YOUR REACH WITH SHOULDER EXERCISES FOR STROKE RECOVERY

Recovering your arm and shoulder movement after a stroke can be challenging. If you can't easily grasp and release objects, move your arms forward, or use your arms to support your weight, it's important to incorporate helpful shoulder exercises for stroke recovery into your daily routine at home.

And that's exactly what Occupational Therapist Hoang Tran recommends. Hoang focuses on shoulder and arm mobility at her outpatient rehabilitation center, Hands-on Therapy. She opened the Florida center in 2014 after extensive clinical experience, including more than a decade at Miami Beach's Mount Sinai Medical Center. As a Certified Hand Therapist (CHT) she specializes in pathological conditions affecting the upper extremities. Throughout her years of working with stroke survivors and other people with upper body trauma, she has learned several simple and effective techniques that you can apply in your own home to speed up your recovery.

SHOULDER EXERCISES FOR STROKE RECOVERY

Hoang knows how crucial it is to expedite your progress as much as possible, and she also understands the importance of supplementing your outpatient therapy with at-home exercises. She recommends the following shoulder exercises for stroke recovery, especially for survivors who lost strength or function in their upper arm.

BASIC-LEVEL SHOULDER EXERCISES

Though strokes are life-threatening and often cause irreversible neurological damage, you may be able to retrain other regions of your brain to make up for this damage. Your muscles must remain active if you hope to use them again, and some exercises aim to achieve this specific task. These two basic-level exercises are recommended for people who still struggle to move or use their shoulder after a stroke.

If you have completely or partially lost function – or even sensation – in one side of your body after your stroke, you still have a very powerful tool at your disposal: the other side of your body. The first exercise will help you use your functioning hand to stretch and stimulate your shoulder muscles. The second focuses on your shoulders themselves, specifically the muscles that allow you to move your shoulder blade on the unaffected side of your body.

1. Towel Slide (Basic)

Get a towel and sit down at a table, desk, or other flat surface. Fold or spread the towel, and make sure it's on the table immediately in front of you. Now, place your affected hand on the towel and put your unaffected hand directly on top of it. Apply enough pressure to keep your hands together, then use your hand to slide the towel away from you, toward the middle of the table.

As your hands move forward, your shoulders will also stretch forward, with the towel reducing friction and allowing your shoulder muscles to stretch and strengthen. If you feel comfortable leaning forward with your upper body, do so in order to slide the towel even farther forward. If you can do this until your arms are almost parallel with your body, the extra movement will allow you to stretch your shoulders at shoulder level, paving the way for a greater range of motion.

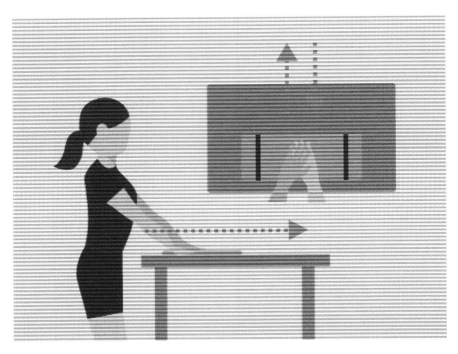

2. Shoulder Shrug

Sit or stand in front of a mirror so that you can clearly see your entire upper body. Now, lift your unaffected shoulder up in a shrugging motion, just as you would if you didn't know the answer to a question. Instead of simply letting it drop again, roll your shoulder back. As you do so, your shoulder blades should get closer together. Repeat this exercise several times each day.

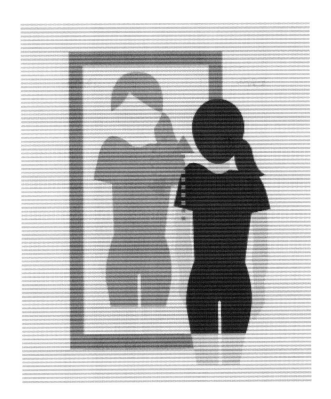

INTERMEDIATE-
LEVEL SHOULDER EXERCISES

These intermediate exercises are ideal if you've already made some progress toward shoulder mobility and control. If you cannot perform them, you may want to continue repeating the basic-level exercises, but don't forget to continue making attempts at these exercises too. They will require a towel, a table, and a cane or any other long, light object.

1. Towel Slides (Intermediate)

This exercise is very similar to the basic-level towel slide, but it incorporates a bigger range of motion by challenging you to stretch your shoulder muscles in more than one direction.

Start by sitting at a table with a towel and placing your affected hand on it, as before. Now use your other hand to slide your hand forward, but don't simply slide it back toward you. Instead, follow this movement by sliding it from side to side. Now slide it back toward you and continue sliding the towel from side to side. Finally, incorporate all of these movements into a series of circular motions, alternating between clockwise and counterclockwise.

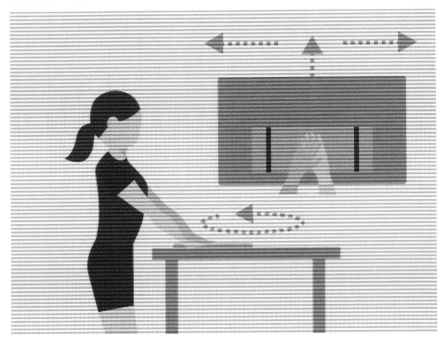

2. External Rotation with Cane

You'll need a cane or lightweight umbrella for this exercise. Hold the cane with both hands in front of your body with your arms bent at a 90-degree angle at your sides. Next, push the cane outward to your left and right without dropping your arms, so that the 90-degree angle remains consistent. This exercise will improve your ability to perform external rotations with your shoulders, which are required for a significant number of everyday tasks.

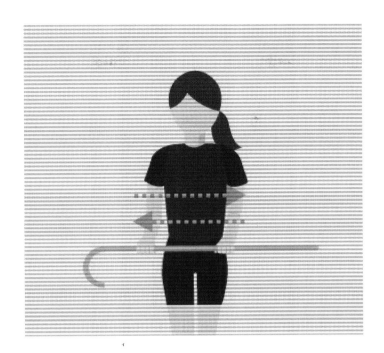

ADVANCED SHOULDER EXERCISES

Finally, a couple of advanced exercises are particularly useful for people who can already grasp objects with their affected hand and move their affected shoulder. If you still haven't regained complete range of motion in both shoulders, but you have enough strength and function to grab and reach in different directions, you may find these helpful. To perform them, you'll need at least five or six cups that can be stacked. Disposable plastic or paper cups are usually the most effective, because they're more lightweight than glasses or hard plastic cups.

1. Behind-the-Neck Cup Pass

Sit at a table and stack the cups right in front of you. Before you begin, remind yourself to keep looking forward throughout the exercise. It may help to train your sights on one specific point ahead of you, such as a painting on the wall or your own reflection in the mirror. Now, grab the first cup from the stack. While continuing to look forward, pass the cup behind your neck and use your other hand to retrieve it and set it back down on the table. Continue doing this until you've passed the entire stack of cups from one hand to the next.

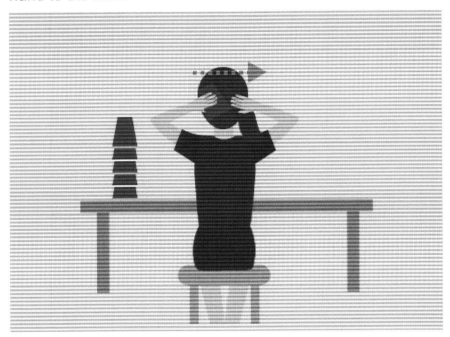

2. Behind-the-Waist Cup Pass

Stand in front of the table, or sit on a stool or backless chair. Re-stack the cups on the table, and bring the first one behind your waist, passing it along the top of your pants line. Retrieve and replace it with the other hand, and repeat.

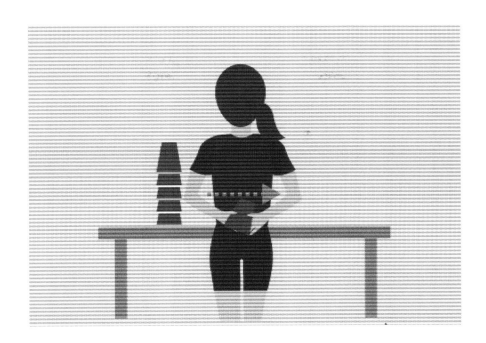

HELPFUL SHOULDER EXERCISES FOR STROKE RECOVERY

The majority of strokes occur in people older than 65, and your risks begin to increase after the age of 55. Survivors can take action to improve their quality of life at any age, so it's important to remain hopeful and proactive instead of assuming the worst. These shoulder exercises for stroke recovery are among the most effective physical therapy techniques, because they tackle the muscles you need the most to regain independence: those in your upper body. If you've suffered from one or more strokes and lost mobility as a result, these exercises will allow you to reclaim control and begin the fulfilling task of retraining your joints and muscles, even after neurological damage.

Published by VAX Books

VaxbookZ.com

Printed in Great Britain
by Amazon